CW00392717

The Ultimate 5:2 Diet Recipe Book

*An Essential Guide to Intermittent Fasting
with Quick and Healthy Recipes incl.
45 Days Weight Loss Challenge and Diet Plan*

1st Edition

Michael Mobson

Our journey to weight loss is not an easy one and some days along the way we need a lot or a little nudge or inspiration to keep us going. Let's say you climb on the scale and the numbers show an increase. The increase is easier to accept when it is well-deserved (it must be those extra calories I pumped in last night!). However, an increase can cause you a lot of frustration when you cannot, for the love of God, figure out a reason for it. Plus, there are days when you are starving, when you feel like you're going to die if you don't eat a calorie-packed, guilt-packed snack, or two.

It's not an easy journey weight loss. You need encouragement because you don't want to let your frustration or cravings win. One way to effectively keep yourself on track is to use a mantra to reinforce your determination. Try to find the one mantra that best suits your purpose and help you fight your "demons". Remember that weight loss is a fight against habits that took years to settle comfortably in your life. Old habits die hard and it takes time to win. You did not put weight on overnight. You can't lose it overnight so be prepared for a long-term lifestyle change. You need to replace old habits with new, healthier ones. Being slender is just the side effect. The real gain and the real purpose of a lifestyle change is getting healthier.

What is the 5:2 diet?

The 5:2 diet is a type of intermittent fasting. As the name properly suggests, intermittent fasting is about alternating non-fasting and fasting periods over a defined period. In the larger sense, fasting has been an essential part of various cultures and religions across the world and practiced successfully for thousands of years. While the motivations behind embracing fasting have changed in time, the result of fasting has remained the same: improved overall health.

The 5:2 diet is, like all intermittent fasting diets, an eating pattern that entails routine fasting. It involves 5 days of normal eating and 2 days of calorie-restricted eating, hence the name. Calorie restriction translates to fewer than 500 Kcal daily for women. For men, it's fewer than 600 Kcal. Made popular by the famous British journalist, Michael Mosley, the 5:2 diet is regarded as a lifestyle more than a proper diet.

The popularity if the 5:2 diet has skyrocketed over the past 10 years mainly due to the numerous success stories that come to back it up. Furthermore, dieters find it easier to stick to than the typical calorie-restricted diets. Why? Simply because this diet does not really restrict **what** you eat, but **when** you eat. During the 2 days that you must restrict your calorie intake to 500 Kcal/day, respectively 600 Kcal/day, you are free to choose what you eat if you respect the calorie restriction. The only real condition is that you **alternate** fasting with non-fasting days, i.e., you need to have at least 1 non-fasting day between the two fasting days.

The 5:2 diet can be a highly effective, easy way to boost metabolism and lose weight. Since it is much easier to oblige than typical calorie-restricted diets, the 5:2 is a diet you would want to consider when you are battling with piling kilos.

How does the 5:2 diet work?

The 5:2 diet works on the same principle as all calorie restricted diets: calorie deficit between calorie intake and calories burnt. You get that calorie deficit during those two fasting days. If done correctly, studies show, not only will you be losing weight, but you are likely to reduce belly fat and maintain muscle mass. Also, as with all diets, the weight loss effects of the 5:2 diet are augmented by practicing exercise, such as strength training or endurance.

The 5:2 diet can, without a doubt, be a very effective weight loss tool **IF** you do not try to compensate the calorie loss from your fasting days during the non-fasting days. Non-fasting days are normal eating days, which means that you must stick to what you would have eaten if you hadn't been fasting. No bonuses. Do not confuse normal eating with eating as much as you can. That is not normal eating. Understand that the 5:2 diet seeks to restrict your calorie intake for 2 days only so that it is easier for you to get that calorie deficit required for weight loss. Let's say you burn 1.500Kcal a day with daily activities and just existing. What that means is that you need to eat maximum 1.500Kcal if you want to maintain your weight. Every calorie you eat above 1.500 Kcal is weight gain. It's all mathematics. You lose weight when you give your body less energy than it consumes. You gain weight when you give your body more energy than it burns.

In a typical calorie restricted died, to lose weight, you need to reduce the 1.500Kcal down to 1.200Kcal/day (for example), i.e., a calorie deficit of 300Kcal per day. In a week, the 300Kcal daily deficit becomes a 2.100Kcal in deficit. With the 5:2 diet, you eat 1.500Kcal every day for 5 days BUT you eat only 500Kcal for 2 days. i.e. your calorie deficit is 1.000Kcal per each day of fasting, i.e., 2.000Kcal per week. The only difference is that it's harder to keep up with a 300Kcal deficit daily that it is with 1.000Kcal deficit for 2 days per week.

Things to pay attention to

Overeating during normal eating days

When your body does not get the calories that it expects, it will ask for more, i.e., you will get hungry. In time, it will get used to it and the days will pass quicker. However, some dieters believe they can overeat in their non-fasting day to compensate for underrating during their fasting days. This approach cancels completely any potential weight loss.

Replacing healthy foods with junk food

Because many dieters get very hungry during the two fasting days, at least in the beginning, they tend to replace the healthier food in their non-fasting days with their junk version. It's like a reward, a reward that, even if it's within the normal calorie limit, it's unhealthy.

Women may experience specific side effects

Some women following the 5:2 diet have experienced one or more missed menstrual periods. However, once they resumed normal eating, this symptom has disappeared. Women, more than men, should stop intermittent fasting if such adverse effects occur.

Certain categories of people should pay attention

The 5:2 diet is a safe diet for the well-nourished, healthy individual. However, there are people that must avoid fasting and dietary restrictions all together, such as

- People suffering or who have been suffering from eating disorders
- Underweight, malnourished, or nutritionally deficient people
- People whose blood sugars level are frequently found dropping
- Teenagers, nursing mothers, pregnant women, children
- People who have been diagnosed with type 1 diabetes
- Women who have fertility issues
- Women who wish to conceive

Benefits of the 5:2 diet

While there are not too many studies conducted to evaluate the 5:2 diet specifically, scientists have dedicated numerous clinical trials and studies to the general concept of intermittent fasting. Without a doubt, this form of dieting benefits our health in many remarkable ways. In addition to the fact that it entails less effort than sticking to an uninterrupted calorie restricted diet plan.

Health benefits of 5:2 diet and intermittent fasting:

- Reduces insulin levels

- Improves insulin sensitivity

- Reduces asthma, heart arrythmias, and seasonal allergies

- Reduces hot flashes during menopause

- Reduces body weight

- Reduces triglycerides levels in the blood

- Reduces fat mass while maintaining muscle mass.

- Decreases levels of leptin

Tips for 5:2 dieters

There is no actual rule to when and what you should eat during the 2 fasting days. Essentially, you need to eat healthy foods if you want to rip the benefits of this diet: lose weight and improved health.

Tips from experienced 5:2 dieters:

- **Adjust the number of meals to your metabolism**
  Some prefer three smaller meals per day, others prefer two slightly bigger meals.

- **Adapt the time you start eating to your own body**
  Some postpone the first meal of the day as late in the day as possible while others need a small breakfast to get them through the day. Simply manage your calories wisely.

- **Focus on nutritious, high-fibre, high-protein foods**
  These foods are not only healthy, but they provide a filling of fullness longer without the added calories.

- **Soups are very efficient to keep you feeling full**
  If you are not a fan of soups, it's time to start exploring the world of soups now. There are plenty of options and variations that you can try. Use quality ingredients and that's it.

- **Mind your portion size and calories**
  It might seem obvious considering how very few calories we are talking about, but the truth is many people get stuck in their habits and stick to eating the same portions. During fasting days, you need to weigh everything and count calories or it will not work.

- **Eat less but use ingredients**
  Examples may include vegetables, plain yogurt, berries, eggs, fish or lean meat. It's better that you use full fat yogurt, but just 1 tbsp. than 2 tbsps. of low-fat, sugar-packed yogurt.

- **Mind the way you cook**
  Lean meat is great if you grill it or boil it, but everything changes if you fry it. The same with veggies: broccoli is amazing, when steamed, but if you cover it oil, you kind of lose the whole purpose of your diet.

However, feel free to experiment! This particular diet allows you to play with the times/number of meals, and type of food until you figure out the combination that works best for you.

Preparation

The 5:2 diet is a calorie restriction diet, even if calorie restriction applies to 2 days out of 7. The first fast days you will most likely face overwhelming hunger. You can counteract the hunger by keeping busy because it tends to go away quickly. Also, because your calorie intake is limited to 25% of a person's normal calorie intake, you may feel slower and weaker.

5:2 dieters said that the fasting days become less challenging and the hunger less overwhelming and they even started looking forward to them after a few weeks. If fasting is not something you are used to, you could keep a snack where you can reach it quickly in case you start feeling faint. However, do not make a habit out of having a snack.

In time, you should stop feeling faint or ill during fasting days so, if this pattern continues, you need to visit your doctor. You may need to end your diet. There are people that simply do not tolerate such low caloric intake, even if it is for two days only.

The 16:8 method

What is it and how does it work?

In addition to the 5:2 diet, the 16:8 method is a form of intermittent fasting that has proven very successful for certain people, hence its popularity. The 16:8 dieters say that it's a suitable, easy, and convenient method to lose weight. First of all, what is the 16:8 method?

As the name properly suggests, 16:8 is about limiting the consumption of food and calorie-containing beverages to the same 8-hour window per day. The remaining 16 hours are fasting hours. You can use this method just 1 day per week or you can use it 7 days per week. It is up to you.

Since it's not as restrictive as other diet plans when it comes to calorie intake and types of food, the 16:8 has become quite popular. It is said to help burn fat, enhance weight loss, prologue life, stabilize blood sugar levels, and boost brain function.

Getting Started with the 16:8 Method

There is no rule as to what the correct or most suitable 8-hour non-fasting window is. You are free to choose whichever 8-hour window suits you best. It's a matter of knowing your body.

- **12 pm to 8 pm:**
  It's best for those who skip breakfast regularly so that they only need to fast overnight. With this window, you can still have a healthy dinner and lunch.

- **9 am to 5 pm:**
  It's for people who need lunch to keep them going and for those who don't have late evening cravings. This window leaves room for a normal lunch and breakfast as well as an early dinner and at least 1 snack.

Irrespective of the window you choose, you must stick to several small meals and snacks so that you keep hunger under control by stabilizing blood sugar levels. Also, it's key that you eat nutritious foods and drink nutritious beverages, not junk food. If you want to get rid of excess weight with the 16:8 method, you can't pack your 8-hour window with 3.000 Kcal worth of junk food just because that's the only time of day you can eat. You must eat your normal calories, just restrict WHEN during the day you are going to it.

Tips for 16:8 Dieters

The two most useful tips that any 16:8 dieter can get is to eat nutrient-rich foods and mind their calorie intake and portions. Variety is key in any diet so including a whole range of whole foods is ideal. Examples may include:

- **Fruits**: Bananas, apples, peaches, berries, etc.
- **Veggies**: Cucumbers, cabbage, cauliflower, broccoli, spinach, tomatoes, etc.
- **Whole grains**: Oats, rice, quinoa, buckwheat, etc.
- **Good fats**: Olive oil, coconut oil, avocados, etc.
- **Protein**: Tofu, meat, fish, eggs, poultry, legumes, nuts, seeds, etc.

Benefits of 16:8 Intermittent Fast

Easy to follow, the 16:8 methods is convenient and flexible. It is also sustainable over longer periods of time. In terms of health, there are many benefits that you must consider:

- **Weight loss** is the most obvious health benefit of this method. Since you only have 8 hours at your disposal to eat, you'll end up consuming fewer calories. Plus, fasting in and by itself has been found to boost metabolism and trigger weight loss.
- 16:8 dieters are also known to manage to **stabilize their blood sugar levels** since fasting lowers blood sugar and reduces insulin levels.

Drawbacks of 16:8 Intermittent Fasting

The main disadvantage of the 16:8 method is a tendency to eat more during the 8-hour eating window to compensate for not eating the remaining 16 hours of the day. Eating too much in such a short window can cause weight gain and trigger unhealthy eating habits and digestive issues.

In terms of short-term effects, fatigue, weakness, and, of course, hunger, are some of the things you should expect after a few days of following the 16:8 diet. When you set into a routine, the hunger, weakness, and fatigue will go away.

There are no studies on humans to support any negative effects on reproductive health, although there are some animal studies that have reported that fasting may interfere with reproduction and fertility in females.

The 16:8 method: is it safe for you?

When you make it a nutritious diet and pair it with a lot of exercise, the 16:8 method can be a very safe, easy, and workable way to shed extra pounds and become healthier. While this method is safe for the average person with no major health issues, there are certain concerns considering people who have suffered or are suffering from eating disorders. Also, individuals who take medicine regularly for certain conditions, people with diabetes that need to eat at regular intervals, or people with low BP (blood pressure) should consult with their physician before embracing the 16:8. Also, women who are dealing with fertility issues, women who are trying to conceive, or women who are breast feeding should not go on intermittent fasting.

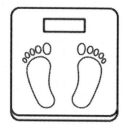

Introduction

This 45-day weight loss plan consists of 45 recipes under 300Kcal that you can adapt and combine in any way you find it suitable so that you get through the 2 fasting days in the 5:2 diet. Also, the recipes have been created in such a way that they are packed with nutrients and the best ingredients and you can easily include them in your 16:8 diet. You can double the smaller portions, or triple in some cases, to get the calorie intake you require for the 8-hour window in the 16:8 method.

Feel free to experiment…

All recipes can be adapted to preference. It is essential that you keep an open mind and substitute ingredients you don't like with the ones you like given that they have similar caloric content. For example, if you don't like spinach, use kale or broccoli or other greens that you like. If you don't have green lentils, use red lentils.

Less is more…

Another important aspect is that you include only healthy ingredients. For example, despite all these recipes being low calorie, you will see the full-fat yogurt included or double cream or whole milk. Well, it's a matter of quality. You don't want the sugars in the low fat, light versions. They are not healthy. It is key that you eat high-quality ingredients. Therefore, even if you need reduce portion size to reach the desired calorie count, stick to good, healthy ingredients.

Cooking is for everyone…

Cooking can be simple if you stick to simple recipes. Remember that you don't need to be a chef to make a soup or a salad from scratch. These are all easy recipes and, while the ingredient list may appear long at times, it's mainly seasonings. Spices add flavour and make the blandest ingredient tasty. Again, feel free to try new combinations! Just make sure you read the instructions carefully and you have everything prepared, including necessary equipment. We have included the equipment for each recipe so you can be prepared. It's nothing fancy, just your typical kitchen gear.

Make larger batches…

One way to make a recipe really tasty and calorie-friendly is to cook larger batches. Like, make dinner for 6, divide in portions, save one portion for you (it's a low-calorie portion) and serve remaining 5 portions to your family (a meal will be around 500-600 kcal for normal eaters). Be creative! Use containers to separate food in portions and serve them to preference.

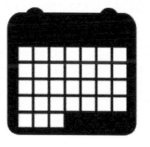

Prep Time: 5 minutes | Cook time: 45 minutes
Skill: Easy | Yields: 6
Nutrition per 1 serving:
Calories: 290.5 | Total Carbs: 28.5 g | Fibres: 4 g
Fat: 7.6 g | Protein: 26.4 g

INGREDIENTS:

♦ 600 g chicken breasts (skinless, boneless)

♦ 150 ml chicken broth

♦ 2 tbsps. olive oil

♦ 6 green onion stalks

♦ 150 g sugar snaps

♦ 150 g tender-stem broccoli

♦ 6 new potatoes (boiled, circa 125 g each)

♦ 1 lemon (cut in wedges)

♦ Dried oregano to taste

♦ Salt and pepper to taste

Serving suggestion: Greens' salad with lemon juice

PREPARATION INSTRUCTIONS:

1. Pre-heat the oven Gas Mark 6, or 180°C. Set the heat on your stove to moderate. Add the oil to an oven-proof pan and heat until shimmering.

2. Place chicken breasts in the hot oil. Fry for 5 minutes turning halfway. The chicken breasts should have a golden crust. Turn the heat off.

3. Pour chicken stock over the chicken breasts in the pan. Cook in the hot oven for 15 minutes. Remove pan from oven and move the chicken breasts to plates.

4. Add the sugar snaps, broccoli, and boiled potatoes to the same pan. Add the lemon quarters and mix to coat the lemon, tatties, and veggies with the stock. Season with pepper and salt and a sprinkle of dried oregano to your preference.

5. Return the chicken to pan. Cook in the oven for 10 minutes. Veggies and tatties should be tender. Chicken should be cooked completely.

6. Plate and enjoy with a huge greens' salad sprinkled with lemon juice!

Prep Time: 5 minutes | Cook time: 15 minutes
Skill: Easy | Yields: 5
Nutrition per 1 serving:
Calories: 233 | Total Carbs: 13 g | Fibres: 2.8 g
Fat: 14 g | Protein: 11.8 g

INGREDIENTS:

♦ 4 anchovy fillets

♦ 3 tbsps. green pitted olives (sliced)

♦ 6 large tomatoes (coarsely chopped)

♦ 1 kg cleaned mussels (yields 480-500g)

♦ 3 tbsps. high-quality olive oil

♦ 150 ml dry white wine of choice

♦ 6 garlic cloves (minced)

♦ 2 bay leaves

Garnish: Parsley or basil (chopped finely)

Serving suggestion: Grilled ciabatta

Equipment: Large stock pot with lid

PREPARATION INSTRUCTIONS:

1. Set the heat on your stove to moderate-low. Add the oil to a stock pot and heat. Gently add the anchovies and fry until they start to break up (circa 2 mins).

2. Add the tomatoes, minced garlic, and green olives to the anchovies. Stir and cook for an extra 5 mins. Add the bay leaves and wine and simmer for 5 mins more.

3. Tip in the mussels and cover. Set heat to moderate-high. Cook for 5 minutes. Shake pot occasionally.

4. Check that the mussels have all opened. Discard the unopened mussels. Plate the mussels. Decorate with the chopped basil or parsley.

Prep Time: 10 minutes | Cook time: 10 minutes
Skill: Easy | Yields: 4
Nutrition per 1 serving:
Calories: 297 | Total Carbs: 4 g | Fibres: 1.6 g
Fat: 42.8 g | Protein: 11 g

INGREDIENTS:

♦ 2 tsps. groundnut oil

♦ Cornflour, to dust

♦ 4 sea bass fillets (circa 175 g each, patted dry)

♦ 1 tbsp. sesame oil

♦ 1 red chilli matchsticks

♦ 30 g root ginger matchsticks

♦ 8-10 spring onion stalks (sliced finely)

♦ 3 cloves of garlic (minced)

♦ 2 x 200 g pak choi

♦ 4 tbsps. teriyake marinade

Garnish: Lime wedges and parsley (chopped)

Serving suggestion: Steamed brown rice

Equipment: Large pan to accommodate the fish; wok and lid to cover.

PREPARATION INSTRUCTIONS:

1. Place the previously patted dry fish fillets on a cutting board. Use the cornflour to dust the fillets on both sides.

2. Turn the heat on your stove to moderate. Add the groundnut oil to a large pan and heat.

3. Place the sea bass fillets in the shimmering oil, skin-side down. Let fry for 3 mins. Flip and cook for an extra minute.

4. In the meantime, add sesame oil to a wok on moderate heat. Drop the chilli, ginger, and spring onions in the wok. Keep stirring as you sauté for 2 minutes.

5. Grab the minced garlic and add to the wok to cook for 1 min. Transfer the sautéed mixture over the fish in the pan.

6. In the same wok, pour the teriyaki marinade and add the pak choi. Cover with a lid and set heat to high. Cook for 1 min. Serve with the fish, lime wedges and steamed rice.

7. Transfer pak choi to plates and top with the fish. Serve with suggested sidings and garnish with lime wedges.

Prep Time: 10 minutes | Cook time: 1 minute
Skill: Easy | Yields: 1
Nutrition per 1 serving:
Calories: 230 | Total Carbs: 18.6 g | Fibres: 8.1 g
Fat: 8.8 g | Protein: 23.4 g

INGREDIENTS:

♦ Cooking spray (preferably olive oil)

♦ 100 g peeled and cooked prawns (pre-packed)

♦ 50 g avocado flesh (cubed)

♦ 120 g bistro salad

♦ 100 g cherry tomatoes (baby plum variety, halved)

♦ 100 g cucumber with peel (cubed)

♦ ½ red onion (small, chopped or julienned)

♦ Salt and pepper to preference

♦ Lemon juice to preference

Garnish: chopped dill, basil, or parsley

Serving suggestion: crispbread, feta cubes, ciabatta, Brie cheese

PREPARATION INSTRUCTIONS:

1. Heat a wok on moderate heat and spray with cooking oil. Add the prawns and allow 1 minute to fry tossing occasionally.

2. Prepare veggies as per instructions and add to a salad bowl. Top with the hot prawns. Season to taste with salt, pepper, and lemon juice. Mix!

3. Chop your favourite garnish and serve with bread or choose of choice!

Prep Time: 10 minutes | Cook time: 8 minutes
Skill: Easy | Yields: 2
Nutrition per 1 serving:
Calories: 271 | Total Carbs: 17.6 g | Fibres: 2.8 g
Fat: 9.7 g | Protein: 18.7 g

INGREDIENTS:

♦ 265 g green lentils from can (drained, rinsed)

♦ 150 g tomatoes (meaty variety, diced finely)

♦ 4 young spring onion stalks (diced finely)

♦ 100 g pomegranate seeds

♦ 2-3 garlic gloves (minced)

♦ 1 bunch parsley (chopped finely)

♦ 1 ½ tbsp. extra-virgin olive oil

♦ 2 free-range eggs (medium, hardboiled)

♦ Lemon juice to preference

♦ Salt and pepper to preference

Serving suggestion: crispy flatbread

PREPARATION INSTRUCTIONS:

1. Cut the eggs to desired size. Set aside.
2. Place all salad ingredients in a large bowl. Reserve the eggs. Tip in the olive oil and sprinkle with lemon juice to preference. Season to liking. Turn to coat. Divide the salad in two bowls.
3. Top each bowl with half the eggs. Enjoy!

SPINACH SCRAMBLED EGGS

Prep Time: 10 minutes | Cook time: 8 minutes
Skill: Easy | Yields: 2
Nutrition per 1 serving:
Calories: 329 | Total Carbs: 24.7 g | Fibres: 10.5 g
Fat: 20.5 g | Protein: 19.2 g

INGREDIENTS:

♦ 1 yellow onion (small, diced very finely)

♦ 1 tbsp. vegetable oil

♦ 1 garlic clove (minced very well)

♦ 1 tbsp. double tomato concentrate

♦ 400 g spinach (chopped)

♦ Salt and pepper to taste

♦ Fresh dill (chopped to preference)

♦ 1 large egg (large, free range, beaten)

Garnish: Cayenne pepper to preference

Serving suggestion: classic crisp bread thins

Equipment: Medium-sized non-stick pan with lid

PREPARATION INSTRUCTIONS:

1. Turn heat on to moderate. Add oil to a deep pan and place on stove. Add the onion and let cook for half a minute while stirring.

2. Set heat to low and cook for an additional 5 minutes. Tip in the minced garlic and fry for no more than 2-3 minutes while stirring from time to time. Add the chopped spinach and cover pan with lid.

3. Increase heat and let cook for 2 minutes with lid on. When spinach has started to wilt, remove lid. Cook until spinach is completely wilted, for 2-3 minutes.

4. Add tomato concentrate, dill, and salt and pepper. Stir to combine. Cook off all extra liquid. Increase heat to high if needed.

5. Move the spinach to one side. Add egg to the cleared side and scramble, and combine with the spinach.

6. Transfer to a serving bowl and sprinkle with cayenne pepper and more dill! Enjoy!

Prep Time:15 minutes | Cook time: 50 minutes
Skill: Easy | Yields: 8
Nutrition per 1 serving:
Calories: 263.5 | Total Carbs: 31.5 g | Fibres: 6.1 g
Fat: 4.3 g | Protein: 24.8 g

INGREDIENTS:

♦ 1.5 litres chicken stock

♦ Sprigs of thyme or rosemary

♦ Bay leaves

♦ 1 onion (diced finely)

♦ 4 chicken breast halves (skinless, boneless)

♦ 2 celery sticks (chopped finely)

♦ 1 kg mixed winter veg (peeled and chopped finely)

Suggestions: carrots, swede, potatoes, parsnip

♦ 150 g pearl barley

♦ Salt to taste

♦ Black pepper to taste

Garnish: parsley, chopped finely

Serving suggestions: bread of choice

Equipment: medium-sized pot with lid; large non-stick pan

PREPARATION INSTRUCTIONS:

1. Add the stock to a pot and bring to the boil on moderate-high heat. Add the chicken, herbs, and onion. Lower heat, cover, and simmer for 20 mins.

2. Remove chicken from pot and set aside to cool. Remove thyme/rosemary sprigs and bay leaves from pot. Discard.

3. Add the winter veggies and celery to the soup pot. Bring to the boil. Add the barley and bring back to the boil. Lower heat, cover, and simmer for 25 minutes.

4. Meanwhile, shred the chicken breast. Keep warm in an air-tight container or oven until ready to use.

5. When the veggies are tender, season the soup to liking. Transfer to soup bowls. Add the shredded chicken breast on top of each bowl.

6. Garnish the soup with the chopped parsley. Enjoy with your favourite bread!

Prep Time: 5 minutes | Cook time: 10 minutes
Skill: Easy | Yields: 2
Nutrition per 1 serving:
Calories: 229 | Total Carbs: 6 g | Fibres: 1.8 g
Fat: 19.5 g | Protein: 9 g

INGREDIENTS:

- 2 tbsps. extra-virgin olive oil
- 1 meaty tomato (large, cubed coarsely)
- 1 clove garlic (sliced finely)
- 100 g asparagus tips, young (halved)
- 2 free-range eggs (medium)
- Cumin or smoked paprika to preference
- Pepper and salt to taste

Garnish: chopped parsley, dill, basil, coriander, etc.
Serving suggestions: fried halloumi cheese; favourite flatbread
Equipment: medium-sized pot with lid

PREPARATION:

1. Warm oil in pan over moderate heat. Add the asparagus halves and fry for 2 mins. Tip in garlic and cook for one minute. Tip in tomatoes and cook for 2 mins.

2. Clear two hollows in the veggies. Crack the eggs in the hollows and cook to liking with the lid on. Season with salt and pepper and cumin or smoked paprika.

3. Plate the egged tomatoes dish and sprinkle with garnish of choice. Serve with fried halloumi or favourite flatbread. Enjoy!

Prep Time: 5 minutes | Cook time: 4-8h + 30 minutes
Skill: Easy | Yields: 4
Nutrition per 1 serving:
Calories: 279 | Total Carbs: 11.8 g | Fibres: 2.8 g
Fat: 36.8 g | Protein: 9.5 g

INGREDIENTS:

◆ 1 large onion

◆ 1 large apio stock (chopped finely)

◆ 3 medium carrots (sliced moderately thick)

◆ 1 yellow bell pepper (cubed)

◆ 1 large potato (cubed)

◆ ⅔ can chopped tomatoes in juice

◆ 500 g beef roasting joint (lean)

◆ Beef stock

◆ Salt to taste

◆ 2 eggs (large, free-range, beaten)

Garnish: Celery leaves (chopped)

Serving suggestions: Soured cream

Equipment: Slow cooker; medium-sized pot

PREPARATION INSTRUCTIONS:

1. Add the cubed beef to the slow cooker and cover with water. Set to high and cook for 4-6 hours. Or, set to low and cook for 8 -12 hours. Beef should be easy to shred.

2. When the beef is tender enough to be shredded easily, remove from slow cooker and shred with a fork. Strain the liquid yielded and set aside.

3. Add onion, bell peppers, carrots, potatoes, and celery stalks to the pot. Cover with water. Turn heat on to moderate and cook until veggie are tender. Pour more water if needed.

4. Add the shredded beef and chopped tomatoes, and cover with the beef stock. Stir and taste. Adjust salt to preference. Allow the tomatoes to cook on low for 5 mins.

5. Beat the eggs in a small bowl until very well combined. Pour in the pot and stir gently to break. Let cook for one more minute. Turn the heat off.

6. Transfer soup to bowls and top with the chopped celery leaves. Serve hot with a heaped spoon of soured cream! Enjoy!

Prep Time: 15 minutes | Cook time: 30 minutes
Skill: Easy | Yields: 6
Nutrition per 1 serving:
Calories: 451 | Total Carbs: 2 g | Fibres: 0 g
Fat: 36 g | Protein: 26 g

INGREDIENTS:

◆ 1 tbsp. vegetable oil

◆ 1 red onion (large, halved, and sliced)

◆ 1 large yellow pepper (seeds removed, chopped)

◆ 1 large red pepper (seeds removed, chopped)

◆ 2 medium courgettes (cut lengthwise and sliced)

◆ 450 ml vegetable stock (homemade)

◆ 300 g couscous

◆ 16 cherry tomatoes (baby plum tomatoes)

◆ Ground black pepper

Garnish: Parsley leaves (chopped)

Serving suggestions: Butter

Equipment: Roasting tin; heatproof bowl with cover

PREPARATION INSTRUCTIONS:

1. Preheat the oven to Gas Mark 4, 180°C/350°F.

2. In a large bowl, combine the vegetables (peppers, onion, and courgette) with the vegetable oil. Place in oven and roast for 25-30 minutes, flipping halfway.

3. In the meantime, bring the stock to the boil. Add couscous to a heatproof bowl. Pour the stock over the couscous. Give it a stir and cover. Set aside for 10 minutes.

4. When the couscous is done, fluff with a fork. Add the roasted veggies and tomatoes and combine with a spatula. Season with salt and pepper to taste.

5. Return the couscous dish to the oven and give it 5 minutes to warm through. Transfer to bowls and serve with freshly chopped parsley and butter.

Prep Time: 5 minutes | Cook time: 10 minutes
Skill: Easy | Yields: 4
Nutrition per 1 serving:
Calories: 211 | Total Carbs: 8 g | Fibres: 1 g
Fat: 16 g | Protein: 11.5 g

INGREDIENTS:

♦ 1 tbsp. olive oil (extra-virgin)

♦ 1 tsp. paprika (preferably smoked)

♦ 3 cloves garlic (minced thoroughly)

♦ 400 g mushroom (sliced finely, chestnut variety)

♦ 1 tsp. salt

♦ 60 ml double cream

♦ 3 green onion sprigs (sliced finely)

♦ 4 thick slices of bread (preferably whole grain)

♦ 4 poached eggs

Garnish: Green onions thinly sliced

Serving suggestions: Paprika

Equipment: Medium-sized, non-stick pan

PREPARATION INSTRUCTIONS:

1. Warm oil in skillet/pan and set heart to moderate. Add the paprika and garlic and fry gently for 1 minute. Add mushrooms, sprinkle with salt, and sauté for 10 minutes.

2. Tip in double cream. Stir gently. Sprinkle the thinly sliced green onions and stir. Simmer for 30 secs to 1 min. Remove from heat. Set aside.

3. Spray bread slices with olive oil. Toast them in a pan over low heat to preference. Transfer bread slices to plates.

4. Load the bread slices with the creamy mushrooms. Ladle the mushrooms with poached egg. Sprinkle a touch of paprika on top. Decorate with green onions.

5. Enjoy!

Prep Time: 15 minutes | Cook time: 30 minutes
Skill: Easy | Yields: 6
Nutrition per 1 serving:
Calories: 214 | Total Carbs: 8 g | Fibres: 2 g
Fat: 9 g | Protein: 24 g

INGREDIENTS:

- 2 tbsps. olive oil (extra-virgin)

- 4-5 tsps. taco mix

- 450 g prawns (peeled, deveined)

- 1 avocado (large, California type, pitted, cubed)

- 1 head Cos lettuce (chopped coarsely)

- 500 g plum tomatoes (cubed)

- ½ jalapeño, deseeded and finely diced, optional

- ¼ red onion (diced finely)

- Coriander to taste (fresh, leaves only, very finely chopped)

- Salt to taste

- Lime juice to taste

Garnish: toasted sesame seeds

Serving suggestions: flatbread; pita chips; tortilla chips

Equipment: medium-sized frying pan

PREPARATION INSTRUCTIONS:

1. Set heat to moderate-high and warm olive oil in the pan.

2. Put the shrimp into the pan along with the taco seasoning. Mix gently to coat. Sear for 2 minutes. Turn heat off.

3. Combine all salad ingredients in a large bowl. Add the taco shrimp. Season to taste and mix to combine well. Enjoy!

Prep Time: 10 minutes | Cook time: 35 minutes
Skill: Easy | Yields: 8
Nutrition per 1 serving:
Calories: 163 | Total Carbs: 30 g | Fibres: 3 g
Fat: 4 g | Protein: 3 g

INGREDIENTS:

- ◆ 2 tbsps. olive oil (extra-virgin)

- ◆ 4 large leeks (chopped thinly)

- ◆ 1.5-2 l vegetable broth (less for thicker soup, more for a thinner soup)

- ◆ 900 g boiling potato (cubed)

- ◆ 3 cloves garlic (minced finely)

- ◆ 2 fresh thyme sprigs

- ◆ 1 bay leaf

- ◆ Salt and pepper to taste

Garnish: Fresh chives to preference (chopped thinly)

Serving suggestions: Hot sauce to taste; cayenne pepper to preference; croutons

Equipment: deep pan (3l), pot (3l), immersion blender or countertop blender

PREPARATION INSTRUCTIONS:

1. Warm olive oil on moderate heat in a deep pan or pot. Add leeks and turn to coat with oil. Set heat to low, cover, and cook for 10 mins.

2. Uncover pot. Add potatoes, garlic, and vegetable stock. Add bay leaf and thyme. Season with pepper and salt to preference. Set heat to moderate and let come to the boil.

3. Set heat back to low. Cover pot and allow the soup to simmer for 15 minutes. Potatoes should be cooked through and easy to spear with a fork.

4. Remove lid. Remove bay leaf and thyme. Blend the soup with a countertop or immersion blender to desired texture.

5. Transfer soup to serving bowls. Sprinkle with fresh chives and a touch of hot sauce or cayenne pepper. Enjoy!

Prep Time: 10 minutes | Cook time: 35 minutes
Skill: Easy | Yields: 8
Nutrition per 1 serving:
Calories: 53 | Total Carbs: 8 g | Fibres: 2 g
Fat: 2 g | Protein: 1 g

INGREDIENTS:

- ◆ 1 tbsp. vegetable oil

- ◆ 1 celery stalk, large (chopped finely)

- ◆ 1 yellow onion, medium (chopped finely)

- ◆ 3 cloves garlic (minced finely)

- ◆ 2 tbsps. tomato paste

- ◆ 800 g chopped tomatoes in juice (2 cans)

- ◆ 1-1.5 litre vegetable stock

- ◆ 2fresh thyme sprigs

- ◆ Salt and pepper to preference

- ◆ Fresh basil to preference (10 g)

Garnish: Basil (freshly chopped)

Serving suggestions: Croutons; focaccia bread; soured cream;

Equipment: Pot or deep pan; countertop or immersion blender

PREPARATION INSTRUCTIONS:

1. Add oil, garlic, onion, and celery to a pan on moderate-high heat. Cook for 3 mins. Add crushed tomatoes, stock, tomato paste, basil, and thyme. Season to taste.

2. Stir and bring to the boil. Set heat to low, cover, and simmer for 15 minutes. Remove lid and thyme sprig. Remove from heat.

3. Blend the soup with equipment of choice to preferred smoothness (countertop or immersion blender). Let cool for a couple of minutes.

4. Transfer to preferred soup bowls. Decorate with chopped basil. Enjoy!

Prep Time: 10 minutes | Cook time: 10-12 minutes
Skill: Easy | Yields: 4
Nutrition per 1 serving:
Calories: 191.3 | Total Carbs: 31.2 g | Fibres: 9.2 g
Fat: 4.2 g | Protein: 10.7 g

INGREDIENTS:

- 2 cloves garlic (minced)
- 1 small yellow onion (diced finely)
- 3 cm ginger (grated)
- 4 tsps. garam masala mix
- Chili flakes to taste
- Salt to taste
- White pepper to preference
- 1 can chopped tomatoes
- 4 tbsps. full-fat yogurt
- 1 can chickpeas (drained and rinsed)
- 4 tbsps. lentils
- 200g broccoli flowerets
- 100 g spinach (chopped)
- Juice of ½ lemon

Garnish: Fresh coriander or fresh parsley (chopped)
Serving suggestions: Low-fat yogurt; pita chips
Equipment: Deep pan with lid

PREPARATION INSTRUCTIONS:

1. Sauté the garlic and onion in the warm oil for 3 minutes on moderate heat. Stir in the garam masala, ginger, chilli flakes, and salt. Cook on low for 2 mins.

2. Tip in the canned tomatoes and yogurt. Add the lentils, broccoli florets, and chickpeas. Stir to mic and cover. Cook for 5 minutes.

3. Add lemon juice and spinach. Stir and cook for 3 additional minutes. Taste and adjust seasonings to liking. Remove from heat.

4. Transfer to bowls. Enjoy with freshly chopped parsley or coriander!

Prep Time: 5 minutes | Cook time: 0 minutes
Skill: Easy | Yields: 4
Nutrition per 1 serving:
Calories: 181 | Total Carbs: 12.5 g | Fibres: 3.9 g
Fat: 9.3 g | Protein: 13.9 g

INGREDIENTS:

- ◆ 4 x 55 g salmon pieces (smoked)
- ◆ 4 large cucumbers (skin on)
- ◆ 110 g Philadelphia cheese
- ◆ ½ red onion (small, chopped finely)
- ◆ Fresh dill to preference (10 g)

Garnish: N/A

Serving suggestions: N/A

Equipment: N/A

PREPARATION INSTRUCTIONS:

1. Remove ends from cucumber and cut them in half lengthwise. Scoop out seeds. Discard the seeds and ends. Set aside, scooped side up.
2. Combine soft cheese with the dill and red onion in a bowl. Mix gently to form a homogenous mixture.
3. Divide cream cheese mixture and add each cucumber half. Spread evenly and top with equal parts of smoked salmon.
4. Bring the cucumber halves together to close the sandwich. Enjoy!

Prep Time: 5 minutes | Cook time: 4 minutes
Skill: Easy | Yields: 1
Nutrition per 1 serving:
Calories: 255 | Total Carbs: 2.3 g | Fibres: 0 g
Fat: 17.6 g | Protein: 21.1 g

INGREDIENTS:

- ◆ 2 eggs (medium, free-range, beaten, seasoned)

- ◆ 1 slice of Turkey deli ham (20 g)

- ◆ 1 mozzarella ball, sliced (20 g)

- ◆ Freshly chopped chives to taste

Garnish: N/A

Serving suggestions: Brie cheese; flatbread; crispbread; Stilton cheese; stir-fried mushrooms

Equipment: small frying pan with lid

PREPARATION INSTRUCTIONS:

1. Heat pan over moderate heat and spray with cooking spray. Pour the beaten eggs in the pan. Cook for 1 minute.

2. Add the turkey slice and arrange the mozzarella slices evenly on the omelette. Sprinkle the chives on top. Cover, reduce heat, and cook for 2 minutes.

3. Remove lid, uncover, and fold. Cook for 30 seconds on each side. Transfer to a plate and enjoy!

Prep Time: 5 minutes | Cook time: 4 minutes
Skill: Easy | Yields: 2
Nutrition per 1 serving:
Calories: 192 | Total Carbs: 10.7 g | Fibres: 2.5 g
Fat: 4.7 g | Protein: 28.8 g

INGREDIENTS:

♦ 1 red onion (small, diced very thinly)

♦ 200 g tuna steak in brine (drained)

♦ ½ cup pickled (sour) gherkins (finely diced)

♦ 50 g tomatoes (cherry, chopped finely)

♦ 1 bunch parsley (stems removed, chopped finely)

♦ 4 heaped tbsps. Greek yogurt (full fat)

♦ 1tbsps. sugar free ketchup

♦ Pepper to taste

♦ Salt to preference (if needed)

Garnish: N/A

Serving suggestions: Serve on crispbread, cucumber slices, flatbread, pita chips, etc

Equipment: N/A

PREPARATION INSTRUCTIONS:

1. Break the tuna steak into smaller pieces and add to a salad bowl. Add onions, parsley, tomatoes, and pickled gherkins, and give it a quick mix.

2. Pour the yogurt and ketchup and ground black pepper to taste. Mix until well combined. Taste and season with salt to liking.

3. Serve on flatbread, crisp thins, crispbreads, etc! Enjoy!

Prep Time: 5 minutes | Cook time: 1 minute
Skill: Easy | Yields: 2
Nutrition per 1 serving:
Calories: 237 | Total Carbs: 16.4 g | Fibres: 8.4 g
Fat: 5.9 g | Protein: 31.7 g

INGREDIENTS:

- ◆ 1 Romaine lettuce head (chopped coarsely)

- ◆ 100 g cooked prawns (drained of any liquid)

- ◆ 300 g cherry tomatoes (halved)

- ◆ 200 g smoked salmon (cut into pieces)

- ◆ Oregano to taste

- ◆ Pepper to taste

- ◆ 20 sprays olive oil

- ◆ Lemon juice to taste

Garnish: N/A

Serving suggestions: Serve with pita chips or flatbread of choice

Equipment: Large salad bowl

PREPARATION INSTRUCTIONS:

1. Put all ingredients in a large bowl, oregano, included, Spray with olive oil. Season to preference. Add the lemon juice and toss or stir to combine.

2. Taste and adjust seasonings to accommodate your taste. Enjoy!

Prep Time: 5 minutes | Cook time: 10-12 minutes
Skill: Easy | Yields: 1
Nutrition per 1 serving:
Calories: 262 | Total Carbs: 14 g | Fibres: 6.4 g
Fat: 11.2 g | Protein: 28.1 g

INGREDIENTS:

- ½ salmon fillets (120g)

- 1 tbsp. capers

- 1 tsp. olive oil

- 2 cloves garlic (very well minced)

- 205 g canned green beans (drained)

- Salt and pepper to taste

Garnish: Chopped parsley

Serving suggestions: Lemon wedges

Equipment: Non-stick pan with lid

PREPARATION INSTRUCTIONS:

1. Heat the pan on moderate and spray with cooking oil. Add the salmon fillet, skin side down. Sear for 1 minute on each side. Turn heat down to low.

2. Add the capers and cover the pan. Cook for 2-3 more minutes until the salmon flakes easily. Remove salmon from pan and onto a plate. Top with the capers.

3. Add olive oil, green beans, and minced garlic to the same pan. Season to taste. Stir to combine. Cook covered for 4-5 minutes on moderate heat.

4. When the green beans are tender, transfer to the plate with the salmon. Drizzle with the juices from the pan. Enjoy with lemon wedges and chopped parsley!

LEMONY ASPARAGUS STIR FRY

Prep Time: 5 minutes | Cook time: 10-12 minutes
Skill: Easy | Yields: 2
Nutrition per 1 serving:
Calories: 206 | Total Carbs: 3 g | Fibres: 0 g
Fat: 6 g | Protein: 33 g

INGREDIENTS:

♦ 1 tbsp. olive oil (extra virgin)

♦ 2 chicken breasts (sliced thinly)

♦ Salt and pepper to preference

♦ 1 tbsp. minced garlic

♦ 100g asparagus tips

♦ Zest of ½ lemon

♦ Juice of ½ lemon

♦ 3 tbsps. soy sauce

Garnish: Lemon zest

Serving suggestions: Steamed brown rice

Equipment: Pan with lid

PREPARATION INSTRUCTIONS:

1. Warm oil in a pan over moderate heat. Add chicken breasts. Sear for 1 min. Season with salt and pepper and sear for 1 additional minute.

2. Add the minced garlic and cover with a lid. Cook for 2 minutes. Remove lid and add lemon juice, asparagus tips, and lemon zest next to the chicken.

3. Cover and cook for 2 minutes. Remove lid and add the soy sauce. Cover and cook for 2 more minutes until the asparagus is tender and the chicken has cooked through.

4. Transfer to plates and serve with lemon zest and steamed rice!

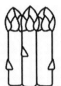

Prep Time: 5 minutes | Cook time: 20-25 minutes
Skill: Easy | Yields: 1
Nutrition per 1 serving:
Calories: 181 | Total Carbs: 13 g | Fibres: 5 g
Fat: 14 g | Protein: 3 g

INGREDIENTS:

- 1 sweet potato (small, peeled, cubed)

- 1 lemon (seeds removed, sliced)

- 360 g green beans (fresh, trimmed)

- 1 tbsp. olive oil

- ½ tsp. salt

- 1 clove garlic (minced)

- ¼ tsp. pepper

- 1 tbsp. fresh rosemary (chopped very finely)

- 1 tbsp. fresh thyme (chopped very finely)

- 1 chicken breast (boneless, skinless)

- ¼ tsp. paprika

- Salt and pepper to taste

Garnish: N/A

Serving suggestions: Lemon juice; steamed rice; couscous;

Equipment: Oven-proof tray

PREPARATION INSTRUCTIONS:

1. Turn oven on and set to Gas Mark 4, 190°C, or 375°F.

2. Add the lemon, sweet potatoes, and green beans to an oven-proof tray previously coated with baking sheet.

3. Drizzle with olive oil. Sprinkle with thyme, rosemary, garlic, salt, and pepper. Use your hands to combine until veggies are well coated. Spread evenly.

4. Add the chicken breast to the tray on top of the veggies. Season with paprika, and salt and pepper. Transfer to oven and bake for 20-25 minutes.

5. When the chicken is cooked and veggies are tender, transfer to a plate and enjoy with more lemon juice!

Prep Time: 5 minutes | Cook time: 16-20 minutes
Skill: Easy | Yields: 4
Nutrition per 1 serving:
Calories: 305 | Total Carbs: 6 g | Fibres: 2 g
Fat: 11 g | Protein: 44 g

INGREDIENTS:

- 3 cloves garlic (minced)

- 2 tbsps. olive oil

- 2 tsps. spice blend of choice

- 410 g chopped tomatoes (canned)

- 60 ml white wine (dry)

- 3 bay leaves (dry or fresh)

- Salt and pepper to taste

- 600 g (4 x 150g) white fish fillets (skin removed)

Suggestions: halibut, cod, or sea bass

Garnish: Basil (fresh, chopped very finely)

Serving suggestions: Lemon juice; steamed rice; couscous.

Equipment: Deep pan with lid

PREPARATION:

1. Pour olive oil in a large pan and set heat to moderate-low. Add ½ of the spice blend and garlic. Cook for 3 minutes while stirring.

2. Turn heat up to moderate. Dump the tomatoes in the pan along with the wine. Add the bay leaves, stir, and let the sauce come to the boil.

3. When the sauce is boiling, turn heat down to low. Let it simmer gently for 5 minutes. Season to taste with the pepper and salt and remaining spice blend. Stir.

4. Grab the fish fillets and place in the sauce. Cover with a lid and let simmer very gently for 6-8 minutes. The fish should begin to flake and turn opaque.

5. When the fish has cooked through, place each fillet in a flat-bottom bowl, ladle with the savoury tomatoes sauce. Serve with basil, very thinly sliced! Enjoy!

Prep Time: 5-10 minutes | Cook time: 0 minutes
Skill: Easy | Yields: 3 |
Nutrition per 1 serving:
Calories: 241 | Total Carbs: 17.7 g | Fibres: 9.1 g
Fat: 10.6 g | Protein: 23.4 g

INGREDIENTS:

- 200 g rotisserie chicken (breast meat only, cubed)
- Chipotle powder to taste
- 20 sprays olive oil
- 1 head Cos lettuce (chopped)
- 2-3 green onion stalks (whole, julienned)
- 1 large avocado (circa 130g, pitted, sliced very finely)
- 150g tomatoes (baby plum variety, halved)
- 85 g sweetcorn (caned)
- Fresh coriander to taste (chopped finely)
- Lemon juice to taste
- Salt and pepper to taste

Garnish: Toasted pumpkin seeds; chia seeds; chopped almonds or pistachio nuts.

Serving suggestions: Flatbread; crispbread;

Equipment: Large salad bowl

PREPARATION INSTRUCTIONS:

1. Add the cubed, shredded rotisserie chicken to a bowl. Spray with olive oil, add a dash of lemon juice, and sprinkle with chipotle powder to taste. Stir to combine.

2. In a large salad bowl, add all salad Ingredients: lettuce, avocado, tomatoes, green onions, sweet corn, and coriander. Salt and pepper to taste. Mix to combine.

3. Taste and adjust seasonings to your preference! Enjoy with garnish and side dish of choice!

Prep Time: 5 minutes | Cook time: 10 minutes
Skill: Easy | Yields: 2
Nutrition per 1 serving:
Calories: 247 | Total Carbs: 21 g | Fibres: 4.6 g
Fat: 11 g | Protein: 13.5 g

INGREDIENTS:

- ◆ 2 large free-range eggs (poached)

- ◆ 1 tbsp. olive oil

- ◆ 4 medium scallions (tops and bulb, diced finely)

- ◆ 300 g shiitake mushrooms (sliced)

- ◆ Salt and pepper to preference

- ◆ Cayenne pepper to preference (optional)

- ◆ Fresh parsley to preference

- ◆ 4 roasted bell peppers (jarred)

Garnish: More parsley, chopped

Serving suggestions: N/A

Equipment: Medium-sized pan

PREPARATION INSTRUCTIONS:

1. Turn heat on to moderate. Warm olive oil in a pan and add the scallions. Stir and cover. Cook for 2 minutes. Turn heat up to moderate-high.

2. Add the mushrooms. Season with cayenne pepper, salt, and pepper. Stir in the parsley. Cook uncovered until all liquid has evaporated stirring occasionally. Transfer to plates.

3. Remove the roasted bell peppers from jar and drain. Slice to preference. Add to plates next to the shiitake mushrooms. Top with freshly chopped parsley.

4. Add one poached egg to each plate. Sprinkle with cayenne pepper. Enjoy!

Prep Time: 5 minutes | Cook time: 8 minutes
Skill: Easy | Yields: 2
Nutrition per 1 serving:
Calories: 272 | Total Carbs: 15 g | Fibres: 5 g
Fat: 12 g | Protein: 25 g

INGREDIENTS:

- 250 g cod fillets (skinless, 2 fillets)

- Lime zest and juice to taste

- Freshly ground black pepper

Salsa Ingredients:

- 1 avocado (small, pitted, diced)

- 2 peaches (stoned and diced)

- 160 g cherry tomatoes (quartered)

- ¼ English cucumber (peel on, diced)

- 2 scallions (tips and bulb, sliced thinly)

- 1 red chilli (deseeded and sliced thinly)

- Fresh coriander to taste (chopped finely)

- Lime zest and juice to taste

- Salt and pepper to taste

Garnish: N/A

Serving suggestions: N/A

Equipment: Ovenproof dish

PREPARATION INSTRUCTIONS:

1. Turn oven on and set to Gas Mark 6 or 200°C.

2. Place the cod fillets in the baking tray. Season with salt and pepper. Sprinkle with lime zest. Drizzle with lime juice to preference.

3. Transfer to the hot oven and bake for 8 minutes. When the fish should flake easily but still retains its moistness, remove from oven and set aside.

4. In a salad bowl, add the salsa ingredients, including lime zest and juice to taste. Season and mix until well combined.

5. Transfer half the salsa onto plates. Top with the baked code fillets. Drizzle with the juices from the baking dish. Enjoy!

Prep Time: 15 minutes | Cook time: 25 minutes
Skill: Easy | Yields: 2
Nutrition per 1 serving:
Calories: 284 | Total Carbs: 19 g | Fibres: 9 g
Fat: 9 g | Protein: 27 g

INGREDIENTS:

- 2 handfuls rocket leaves

- 175 g green beans (trimmed)

- 2 x 120 g beef sirloin (fat removed, beaten to 4 mm thickness,)

Marinade:

- 1 tbsp. balsamic vinegar

- 2 tsp. thyme leaves

- 1 finely grated garlic clove

- 1 tsp. rapeseed oil

- Black pepper to taste

Warm salad:

- 1 sliced garlic clove

- 1 tsp. rapeseed oil

- 2 red onions (sliced julienne)

- 2 cooked beetroot (wedged)

- 6 pitted green olives (quartered)

Garnish: N/A

Serving suggestions: N/A

Equipment: Steamer, non-stick frying pan

PREPARATION INSTRUCTIONS:

1. Mix the marinade ingredients in a bowl. Add the steaks to the bowl and combine. Set aside. Steam the green beans until just tender (4-6 mins). Transfer to plates.

2. Add oil to a non-stick skillet and warm on moderate heat. Add the garlic slices and onions and sauté for 8-10 minutes. Push mixture to one side.

3. Add the steaks to the cleared side of the pan. Sear on each side for 3 minutes to a medium-rare doneness. Pile the steaks on top of the steamed green beans.

4. To the same pan, add the beetroot, olives, and marinade. Cook to warm through. Transfer mixture around and on steaks. Place the rocket next to it. Enjoy!

Prep Time: 10 minutes | Cook time: 20 minutes
Skill: Easy | Yields: 4
Nutrition per 1 serving:
Calories: 262.5 | Total Carbs: 37.7 g | Fibres: 5.8 g
Fat: 9.8 g | Protein: 7.9 g

INGREDIENTS:

- ♦ 170 g dry quinoa(cooked)
- ♦ 300 g meaty tomatoes (diced finely)
- ♦ 300 g cucumber (diced)
- ♦ 1 yellow bell pepper (diced)
- ♦ 1 orange bell pepper (diced)
- ♦ 1 large bunch parsley (chopped)
- ♦ 2 tbsps. extra virgin olive oil
- ♦ Lemon juice to taste
- ♦ Salt and pepper to taste

Garnish: More parsley

Serving suggestions: Pita chips

Equipment: N/A

PREPARATION:

1. Add all ingredients to a large bowl. Season with salt and pepper. Mix well until well combined. Taste and add lemon juice to taste.

Prep Time: 5 minutes | Cook time: 5-10 minutes
Skill: Easy | Yields: 4
Nutrition per 1 serving:
Calories: 237 | Total Carbs: 3 g | Fibres: 1 g
Fat: 20 g | Protein: 12 g

INGREDIENTS:

- 2 tbsps. extra-virgin olive oil

- 1 sprig rosemary (chopped)

- 1 250g-pack halloumi cheese (bite-size chunks)

- 1 red onion (small, cut into 8 wedges)

- 1 courgette (ends trimmed, cut into 8 pieces)

- 4 lemon wedges (cut into halves)

- Salt and pepper to preference

Garnish: N/A

Serving suggestions: Houmous; couscous

Equipment: Metallic skewers; glass bowl with lid; barbecue/oven with grill function

PREPARATION INSTRUCTIONS:

1. Mix olive oil, lemon zest, lemon juice, and rosemary in a glass bowl. Add the halloumi and coat with the marinate. Cover and set aside for 15 mins.

2. Thread halloumi, lemon wedges, red onion, and courgette onto skewers. Barbecue or grill in the oven for 5-10 mins while brushing occasionally with leftover marinade.

3. Transfer to plates and enjoy!

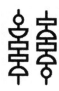

Prep Time: 5 minutes | Cook time: 10-15 minutes
Skill: Easy | Yields: 4
Nutrition per 1 serving:
Calories: 287 | Total Carbs: 27 g | Fibres: 2 g
Fat: 9 g | Protein: 25 g

INGREDIENTS:

- Cooking oil spray

- 450 g raw prawns (peeled and deveined)

- Salt and pepper to preference

- 1 tsp. garlic (minced)

- 85 g honey

- Juice of 1 lemon

For the stir-fry:

- Cooking oil spray

- 450 g asparagus tips (halved)

- 1 red bell pepper (cut into matchsticks)

- 1 tsp. garlic (minced)

- Salt and pepper to preference

Garnish: Fresh parsley (chopped finely)

Serving suggestions: Steamed brown rice

Equipment: Non-stick skillet, medium-sized;

PREPARATION INSTRUCTIONS:

1. Spray a non-stick frying pan with cooking oil and heat on moderate heat. Add prawns, garlic, lemon juice, and honey. Season to taste. Stir well and cook for 4 minutes turning halfway. Prawns should be opaque and pink. Remove from heat.

2. Meanwhile, spray another skillet with cooking oil and heat on moderate heat. Add the asparagus, garlic, and bell pepper matchsticks. Season to taste. Cook to preferred doneness. Remove from heat and transfer to a large bowl.

3. Add the prawns to the same bowl. Stir to combine. Taste and adjust seasonings if needed! Serve with chopped parsley and desired side!

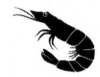

Prep Time: 5 minutes | Cook time: 8 minutes
Skill: Easy | Yields: 1
Nutrition per 1 serving:
Calories: 249.4 | Total Carbs: 25.2 g | Fibres: 6 g
Fat: 12 g | Protein: 12.3 g

INGREDIENTS:

- ◆ 1 slice seeded bread

- ◆ 1 extra-large egg (hardboiled, sliced lengthwise)

- ◆ 25 g houmous (divided)

- ◆ 1 small tomato (sliced)

Garnish: Cayenne pepper or smoked paprika for the houmous.

Serving suggestions: Greens salad drizzled with lemon juice.

Equipment: N/A

PREPARATION INSTRUCTIONS:

1. Spread half of the houmous on the slice of seeded bread. Top with the egg slices.

2. Spread remaining houmous on top of the egg slices. Top with tomato slices.

3. Enjoy!

Prep Time: 5 minutes | Cook time: 0 minutes
Skill: Easy | Yields: 1
Nutrition per 1 serving:
Calories: 268 | Total Carbs: 47.2 g | Fibres: 6.9 g
Fat: 6.4 g | Protein: 10.2 g

INGREDIENTS:

- 40 g soba noodles (cooked from dry)
- 150 g cherry tomatoes (halved)
- 1 tbsp. mashed avocado
- 1 tbsp. chia seeds
- 28 g cooked quinoa
- Juice of ½ lemon or more
- Salt and pepper to taste

Garnish: Chopped fresh parsley

Serving suggestions: Flatbread of choice

Equipment: N/A

PREPARATION INSTRUCTIONS:

1. Mix the salad ingredients in a bowl and season with salt and pepper. Adjust lemon juice to preference. Top with fresh parsley and enjoy!

Prep Time: 5 minutes | Cook time: 0 minutes
Skill: Easy | Yields: 4
Nutrition per 1 serving:
Calories: 172 | Total Carbs: 3 g | Fibres: 0 g
Fat: 7 g | Protein: 23 g

INGREDIENTS:

- ◆ 40 g Greek yogurt

- ◆ 1 avocado (mashed)

- ◆ 1 tbsp. lemon juice

- ◆ 1 garlic clove (minced)

- ◆ Salt and pepper to taste

- ◆ 250 g chicken breast (cooked and cubed)

- ◆ 50 g celery stalks (diced finely)

- ◆ ½ large red onion (diced finely)

- ◆ 2-3 slices jalapeño (diced finely)

- ◆ Fresh parsley (chopped)

Garnish: Sriracha sauce

Serving suggestions: Bread of choice

Equipment: N/A

PREPARATION INSTRUCTIONS:

1. In a large bowl, add the avocado, minced garlic, and yogurt. Season to taste with pepper and salt. Combine to a homogenous consistency. Add lemon juice to taste.

2. Dice the onions, jalapeño, parsley, and celery and add to the avocado and yogurt bowl. Add the cubed chicken breast. Combine well.

3. Serve on favourite bread/toast or drizzled with sriracha or barbecue sauce! Enjoy!

Prep Time: 5 minutes | Cook time: 60 minutes
Skill: Easy | Yields: 6
Nutrition per 1 serving:
Calories: 181 | Total Carbs: 16.2 g | Fibres: 4.9 g
Fat: 6.9 g | Protein: 15.5 g

INGREDIENTS:

♦ 2 tbsps. vegetable oil

♦ 250 g lean steak mince, 5% fat

♦ 1 large yellow onion (chopped)

♦ 1 medium yellow bell pepper (diced)

♦ 1 large carrot(julienned)

♦ 1 tsp. ground cumin

♦ 1 tsp. cayenne pepper

♦ ½ tsp. ground coriander

♦ Salt and pepper to taste

♦ 250 ml beef stock

♦ 1 bay leaf

♦ 1 can chopped tomatoes

♦ 1 can mixed bean salad in water (drained, rinsed)

♦ Jalapeno slices to taste (chopped finely)

Garnish: Fresh parsley (chopped)

Serving suggestions: Topped with poached eggs and served with tortilla chips.

Equipment: Medium-sized wok or deep pan

PREPARATION INSTRUCTIONS:

1. Add oil to the wok and heat on moderate heat. Add the onions, carrots, and bell peppers and cook for 5 minutes. Add seasonings and turn to coat.

2. Add the minced beef and cook until browned, stirring occasionally to break it into smaller grains. Add beef stock and bay leaf and stir to combine. Cook for 5 mins.

3. Add the chopped tomatoes, mixed beans, and jalapeno. Bring to the boil. Lower heat and simmer until the chilli has reduced to desired consistency.

4. Taste and adjust seasonings accordingly. Plate and top with fresh parsley. Top with poached egg or grated cheddar cheese. Enjoy!

Prep Time: 5 minutes | Cook time: 60 minutes
Skill: Easy | Yields: 6
Nutrition per 1 serving:
Calories: 451 | Total Carbs: 2 g | Fibres: 0 g
Fat: 36 g | Protein: 26 g

INGREDIENTS:

- ◆ 10 olive oil sprays
- ◆ 1 small chicken breast (120 g)
- ◆ 1 to 1½ tsp. Cajun spice blend
- ◆ Lemon juice to taste
- ◆ 200 g green beans (canned, drained, rinsed)
- ◆ Salt and pepper to preference

Garnish: N/A

Serving suggestions: N/A

Equipment: Non-stick skillet with lid & griddle pan; kitchen rolling pin

PREPARATION INSTRUCTIONS:

1. Beat the chicken with a rolling pin to 1-cm thickness. Spray with the olive oil, sprinkle the Cajun spice blend, and drizzle with lemon juice. Coat on all sides.

2. Heat griddle on moderate-high heat. When hot, put the chicken breast on and cook on both sides to preference. Remove from heat and transfer to a plate.

3. Heat a pan over moderate heat and add the canned beans. Cover with lead and cook for 4-6 minutes or as instructed on the can. Season to taste. Add to the plate with the chicken. Enjoy!

Prep Time: 5 minutes | Cook time: 15 minutes
Skill: Easy | Yields: 6
Nutrition per 1 serving:
Calories: 136 | Total Carbs: 0 g | Fibres: 0 g
Fat: 8 g | Protein: 12 g

INGREDIENTS:

- ◆ Cooking oil spray (6 sprays)

- ◆ 480 ml egg white (mixed to a fluid consistency)

- ◆ 1 tomato (diced)

- ◆ 80 g spinach (chopped)

- ◆ Pickled jalapeños to taste (chopped finely)

- ◆ Salt and pepper to taste

Garnish: N/A

Serving suggestions: Grated parmesan cheese

Equipment: 6-cup muffin tray

PREPARATION INSTRUCTIONS:

1. Turn oven on and set to Gas Mark 5, 180°C, or 350°F.

2. Spray the muffin tray with cooking spray and use a brush to coat each cup with the oil. One spray per cup should be enough.

3. Place equal amounts of spinach, tomatoes, and jalapeno in each cup.

4. Mix egg whites to a fluid consistency. Season with salt and pepper. Pour over the veggie cups.

5. Place in the oven and cook until the eggs whites have become opaque, circa 15 minutes. Remove from oven and transfer to plates. Enjoy!

Prep Time: 5 minutes | Cook time: 0 minutes
Skill: Easy | Yields: 1
Nutrition per 1 serving:
Calories: 201.5 | Total Carbs: 7.8 g | Fibres: 4.1 g
Fat: 16 g | Protein: 8.1 g

INGREDIENTS:

- ◆ 1 large egg (hardboiled egg, cubed)

- ◆ 28 g pitted green olives (small variety)

- ◆ 1 small tomato (circa 90g, cubed)

- ◆ 35 g avocado (diced or sliced finely)

- ◆ Salt and pepper to taste

Garnish: Fresh parsley (chopped)

Serving suggestions: Snack, or next to fried chicken breast

Equipment: Small salad bowl

PREPARATION INSTRUCTIONS:

1. Add all salad ingredients, i.e. avocado, tomatoes, egg, and green olives to a bowl. Season with pepper and salt to your preference. Mix and serve!

Prep Time: 5 minutes | Cook time: 0 minutes
Skill: Easy | Yields: 1
Nutrition per 1 serving:
Calories: 237 | Total Carbs: 44 g | Fibres: 7 g
Fat: 3 g | Protein: 9 g

INGREDIENTS:

- 40 g black or red kidney beans (canned)

- 2 tbsps. sweetcorn

- 40 g cooked quinoa

- 1 garlic clove (minced)

- ½ large red onion (diced)

- Fresh cilantro to taste

- Lime juice to taste

- Salt and pepper to taste

Garnish: N/A

Serving suggestions: Snack or next to eggs

Equipment: Small bowl

PREPARATION:

1. Add all salad ingredients, i.e. avocado, tomatoes, egg, and green olives to a bowl. Season with pepper and salt to your preference. Mix and serve!

Prep Time: 5 minutes | Cook time: 0 minutes
Skill: Easy | Yields: 4
Nutrition per 1 serving:
Calories: 144 | Total Carbs: 12 g | Fibres: 3 g
Fat: 7 g | Protein: 7 g

INGREDIENTS:

- ◆ 4 tsp. pesto

- ◆ 4 tbsps. crumbled feta cheese

- ◆ 260 g canned chickpeas (drained and rinsed)

- ◆ 260 g cherry tomatoes (quartered)

Garnish: N/A

Serving suggestions: Snack or next to grilled turkey or chicken

Equipment: Medium-sized salad bowl

PREPARATION:

1. Add all salad ingredients, i.e. avocado, tomatoes, egg, and green olives to a bowl. Season with pepper and salt to your preference. Mix and serve!

Prep Time: 5 minutes | Cook time: 0 minutes
Skill: Easy | Yields: 2
Nutrition per 1 serving:
Calories: 233 | Total Carbs: 19.2 g | Fibres: 9.9 g
Fat: 16.8 g | Protein: 4.4 g

INGREDIENTS:

- 210 g avocado flesh

- 150 g cherry tomatoes (diced as finely as you can)

- 1 red onion (small, diced very finely)

- 1 canned jalapeno pepper (diced finely)

- 3 garlic cloves (minced)

- 1 bunch parsley (finely chopped)

- Lemon juice to taste

- Salt and pepper to taste

Garnish: N/A

Serving suggestions: Snack or next to grilled turkey or chicken

Equipment: Mortar and pestle; salad bowl

PREPARATION:

1. Add the avocado to the mortar and mash with the pestle to a rough consistency. Transfer to the salad bowl. Add the garlic to the same mortar and mince. Transfer to bowl over the avocado.

2. Add the jalapeno, parsley, red onion and tomatoes to the same bowl. Season with pepper and salt to taste. Mix to combine. Taste and adjust lemon juice to preference! Enjoy!

Prep Time: 10 minutes | Cook time: 16 minutes
Skill: Easy | Yields: 4
Nutrition per 1 serving:
Calories: 238
Total Carbs: 34 g
Fibres: 5 g
Fat: 7 g
Protein: 11 g

INGREDIENTS:

- ◆ 2 tsp. cumin seeds
- ◆ 1 tsp. chilli flakes
- ◆ 2 tbsps. olive oil
- ◆ 140 g split red lentils
- ◆ 600 g carrots (washed, peeled, grated)
- ◆ 125 ml milk
- ◆ 1l vegetable stock (hot)
- ◆ Salt and pepper to taste

Garnish: Fresh parsley (chopped)

Serving suggestions: Plain Greek yogurt, naan bread, pita bread

Equipment: Deep saucepan; stick blender or food processor; pot to warm the veggie stock

PREPARATION INSTRUCTIONS:

1. Toast the chilli flakes and cumin seeds in a saucepan over moderate heat for 1 min. Transfer half to a small bowl and set aside.

2. To the same saucepan, add the olive oil, grated carrots, split red lentils. Pour the hot veggie stock and milk into the pan and bring to the boil.

3. Lower heat and let the soup simmer for 15 mins. When the lentils and carrots have softened, whizz with an immersion blender to preferred smoothness.

4. Season to with pepper and salt to preference. Garnish with chilli flakes and cumin seeds and a sprinkle of chopped parsley. Enjoy!

Prep Time: 5 minutes | Cook time: 0 minutes
Skill: Easy | Yields: 1
Nutrition per 1 serving:
Calories: 162 | Total Carbs: 39.9 g | Fibres: 10.9 g
Fat: 1.3 g | Protein: 2.6 g

INGREDIENTS:

- ◆ 100 g raspberries
- ◆ 100 g blueberries
- ◆ 100 g strawberries (quartered)
- ◆ 1 tsp. honey (optional)
- ◆ 1 tsp. lemon juice (optional)

Garnish: N/A

Serving suggestions: Plain yogurt

Equipment: N/A

PREPARATION INSTRUCTIONS:

1. Add the fruit to a bowl. Mix to combine.
2. Add the honey and lemon juice to another small bowl. Whisk to combine.
3. Pour lemon and honey sauce over the berries! Enjoy!

Prep Time: 5 minutes | Cook time: 0 minutes
Skill: Easy | Yields: 1
Nutrition per 1 serving:
Calories: 252
Total Carbs: 50 g
Fibres: 6.7 g
Fat: 5.6 g
Protein: 6.2 g

INGREDIENTS:

- ◆ 40 g plain muesli

- ◆ 100 ml Alpro Oat Original

- ◆ 1 medium nectarine (sliced finely)

Garnish: N/A

Serving suggestions: Sprinkle with crushed toasted almonds

Equipment: N/A

PREPARATION INSTRUCTIONS:

1. Add the muesli to a small bowl. Warm the milk in the microwave for 30 seconds. Pour over the muesli. Add 50 ml of hot water.

2. Cover with a plate and set aside for 5 minutes until the muesli has swelled. Top with the nectarine slices. Enjoy!

Prep Time: 5 minutes | Cook time: 15-20 minutes
Skill: Easy | Yields: 4
Nutrition per 1 serving:
Calories: 201 | Total Carbs: 5.8 g | Fibres: 2 g
Fat: 12.6 g | Protein: 15 g

INGREDIENTS:

- ◆ Cooking spray

- ◆ 60 g spicy Chorizo sausage (diced)

- ◆ ½ small red onion (julienned)

- ◆ 2 cloves garlic (minced)

- ◆ 2 roasted red pepper (from jar, drained, sliced)

- ◆ 100 g frozen peas

- ◆ 4 large eggs (beaten)

- ◆ 25 g parmesan (grated)

Garnish: Freshly chopped parsley

Serving suggestions: Bistro salad dressed with sherry vinegar

Equipment: Non-stick ovenproof pan

PREPARATION INSTRUCTIONS:

1. Turn oven grill on to high.

2. Spray an oven-proof pan with cooking oil and heat over moderate heat. Add the diced chorizo and fry for 1-2 minutes. Lower heat and add onions. Fry for 5 mins.

3. Stir in garlic and cook until fragrant, circa 2 mins. Stir in the frozen peas and red bell pepper. Pour the eggs onto the chorizo mixture and season to preference.

4. Allow the frittata to cook 2 minutes. Top with the parmesan, pop under the oven grill, and grill until the centre is set and the top has turned golden. Enjoy!

Prep Time: 5 minutes | Cook time: 0 minutes
Skill: Easy | Yields: 2
Nutrition per 1 serving:
Calories: 211 | Total Carbs: 28.5 g | Fibres: 0 g
Fat: 8 g | Protein: 8.5 g

INGREDIENTS:

- 1 tbsp. olive oil

- 200 g garden peas (frozen)

- 1 large carrot (diced

- 270 g canned green beans (drained)

- 1 small yellow onion (small, julienned)

- 3 tbsps. tomato puree

- 1-2 chicken stock cubes

- 250 ml water, or more

- Chopped dill to taste

- Salt and pepper to taste

Garnish: More dill

Serving suggestions: Warm pita

Equipment: Wok or deep pan with lid

PREPARATION INSTRUCTIONS:

1. Heat oil in a wok over moderate heat. Add the onions and carrots and cook for 1 minute. Cover and cook for 8 minutes.

2. Remove lead and add the frozen peas. Cover and cook with lid on for 5-6 minutes. Uncover and add the green beans, tomato puree, stock cubes and water to cover.

3. Cover and cook for 5 minutes with lid on. Uncover and cook until the liquid has cooked off to your preference. Beans and peas should be tender, not mushy.

4. Chop dill and add to the wok. Stir to combine. Season to taste with pepper and salt. Transfer to bowls and enjoy with suggested sides!

Prep Time: 5 minutes | Cook time: 10 minutes
Skill: Easy | Yields: 3
Nutrition per 1 serving:
Calories: 216 | Total Carbs: 25.4 g | Fibres: 5.7 g
Fat: 11.1 g | Protein: 6.8 g

INGREDIENTS:

- 2 tbsps. olive oil

- 3-5 garlic cloves (minced)

- 500 g shiitake mushrooms (sliced)

- 185 g cooked quinoa

- Fresh parsley (chopped)

- Lemon juice to taste

- Salt and pepper to taste

Garnish: Toasted sesame seeds

Serving suggestions: Next to grilled chicken

Equipment: Non-stick frying pan

PREPARATION INSTRUCTIONS:

1. Warm the oil in skillet over moderate-high heat. Add the shiitake mushrooms, season, and stir to combine. Cook for 2 minutes stirring occasionally.

2. Add the minced garlic and stir. Cook for 2 more minutes. Cover and cook for an additional 5 minutes. Remove heat and cook until all liquid has evaporated.

3. Meanwhile, add quinoa and parsley to a bowl. When the mushrooms are ready, add them to the bowl. Stir to combine. Taste and season with salt, pepper, and lemon juice as per preference.

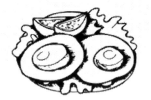

Printed in Great Britain
by Amazon